10 Minute Workout
40 Interval Workouts You Can Do Anytime and Anywhere

Table of Contents

Introduction

You have a tight schedule to stay on, after all you have to get your kids to school, to soccer, and back home again, and you need to get your own work done at the office. Don't even mention the errands you have to do and the house you have to keep. At the end of the day, when you catch a glimpse of yourself in the mirror, you remember the gym was on your to-do list today.

Just like it was yesterday and the day before, but somehow you just can't manage to squeeze in that hour or two to get down there and run on a treadmill for a bit. You tell yourself you will do better next week, but your days are the same day in and day out, and you are left wondering when you are ever going to lose that extra few pounds that has been hanging on.

"I'm busy"

"I don't have time"

"I am too tired to go out again"

"Gym memberships are expensive"

Everything you tell yourself that keeps you out of the gym and in the shape you are in right now. Of course it's true. You are tired, you do work hard, and you do have a lot to do already. If you are living life on a budget as most people do, then you probably already don't want to invest in a membership at the gym, too.

Whatever your reason is, you know you have to make a change, and soon. And that is where this book comes in. Using exercises you can do anytime of the day… they only take 10 minutes… and anywhere you want… they use your own body weight… you don't have any more reason to not work out.

Let this book change the way you think about exercise, and get ready to lose the weight and tone up like you have been dreaming of.

Changing your life and getting healthy once and for all has never been so fast and easy to do. You got this.

Chapter 1 – Let's Get Started

Now I don't really thing I need to get into all of the reasons you ought to get healthy. I think it's pretty obvious given the things you know about how you feel right now and how you would feel if you increased your fitness level.

I'm not even saying that you have to lose weight. There are a lot of people that are a normal weight based on what the scale tells them, but they are far from healthy. In order to be healthy, you need to get your heart rate up for a period of time in a day and work out those muscles.

You may find the number on the scale changes a bit, whether you are already skinny and you see it rise as you gain muscle. This is because muscle weighs a lot, and if you aren't very muscular right now and gain some, you will see your weight rise. That is not a bad thing by any means! The goal is to get healthy, and that is just what we are going to do.

If you want to lose weight, you will certainly do that when you start working out with this plan. You will see the weight melt off of you as you work towards your goal, but you will love how it doesn't take you very long to do it. It would have been groundbreaking news back in the day if they knew you could lose the weight you want to lose but only spend a few minutes a day doing it.

I know that sounds crazy when you first hear it, but interval training is a new way of working out, and by doing it, you will see that you can get way healthier and it won't take much time at all. This is because your body responds to the high intensity part of the cardio, then as it recovers you work on sculpting and changing where you need.

The way this works sounds funny, but it really does. For just a few minutes a day you would be amazed by all of the people that have sculpted their bodies into exactly what they want them to be.

You don't have to stress out at the gym, or better yet, even set foot inside of one. In the chapters to come, I am going to show you how you can lose weight and get fit all with your own body, any time, and any place.

Chapter 2 – Bring Your Own Gym: Body Weight Workouts

We are always told to go to the gym, to work out for a few hours, and to use all of these different pieces of equipment. There are a number of issues that arise when you go about losing weight this way. Perhaps you don't have the time to go to the gym, or maybe you don't have the money to go. Maybe you don't want to work out in front of other people, or perhaps you don't feel comfortable in front of other people.

Whatever your reason is, you just don't want to go to the gym. There is good news, however, because you don't have to. You can use your own body weight to work against you, and strengthen your body this way.

As funny as it sounds, you actually can get even better results using your own body weight against yourself to work out than if you were to use weights at the gym. Take a look at these different moves, and combine them into your workout later on!

Push ups

Stand on the balls of your feet with your hands flat on the ground, out to either side of you. As you drop your chest to the floor, your arms will form right angles. Keep your head looking forward.

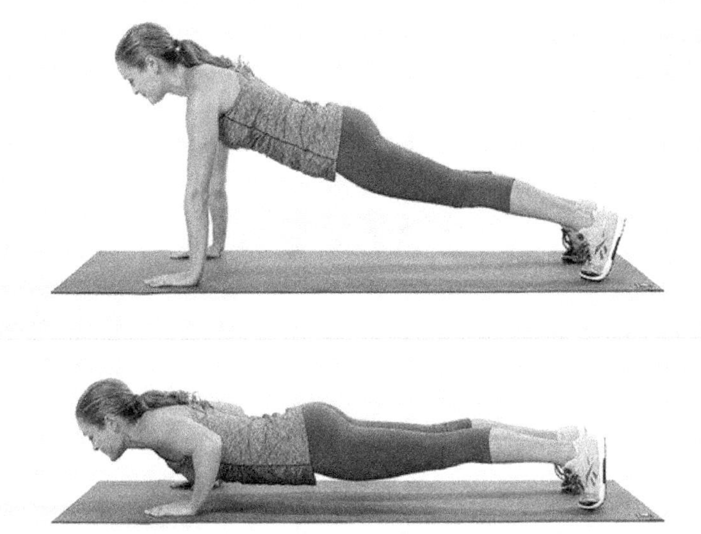

Don't strain it up or look down.

Pull ups

Grab onto a bar above your head, lifting your hands above your head but keep them facing you. Slowly lift your body weight up as high as you can, then slowly lower yourself once more.

Repeat as many times as you can.

Planking

Get on the balls of your feet like you would with a push-up, only instead of having your hands off to either side, keep them directly beneath you.

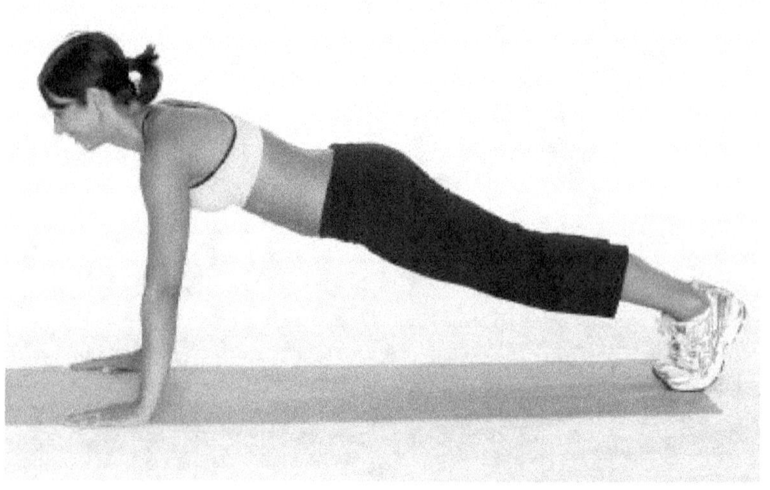

Keep your bottom elevated where it is naturally, don't raise it high or let your back droop down.

Side raises

Lay on your side with your legs out straight and your elbow on the ground. Place your upper hand on your hip, and lift your hip up to the air.

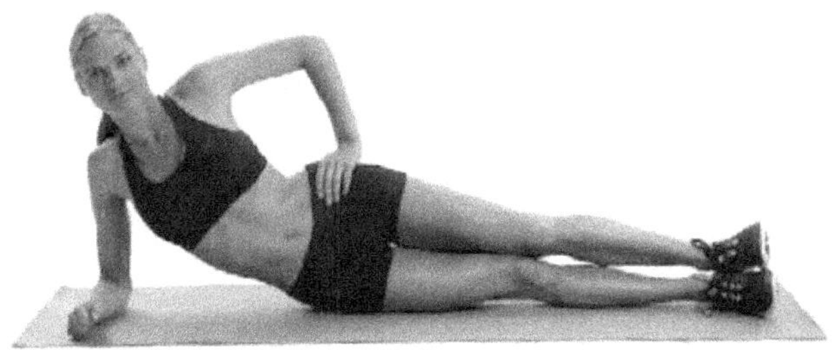

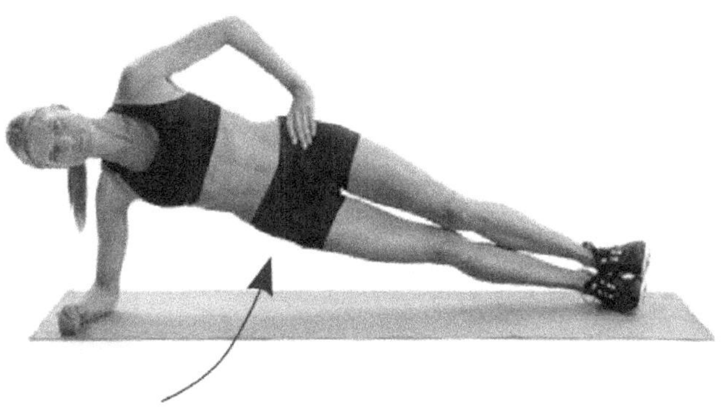

Slowly lower yourself down again; rolling out of your elbow as you lift and settling easily back down.

Walking lunges

Start by standing up straight, and then take a step forward. Sink down and bend your knee into a right angle, only don't let your knee go further forward than your toes.

It's really bad for your knees to go further than your toes, so only go as far as a right angle. As you are settled down, your other leg should be bent as well.

Stand up out of your lunge, and go immediately into your next lunge on the other leg. Make sure you have enough room to do this before you begin, and try doing a few one way and turn around to do a few more the other way.

If you don't have room to move, simply do one lunge, then stand up and do the opposite leg. This is called alternating lunges.

Wall pushups

Stand up facing a wall, with your feet a few feet out into the room. Keep your legs straight, and your feet planted firmly on the floor as you place your hands out to either side of you on the wall.

Lean your weight against the wall, and then push your body weight up until you are at full arm's length. Slowly let yourself fall back down towards the wall. Keep your movement slow and deliberate.

Squats

Stand with your feet slightly wider than your hips. Point your feet forward, and sink your bottom back towards the floor. Keep your back straight and sit back until your knees are at a right angle to the floor.

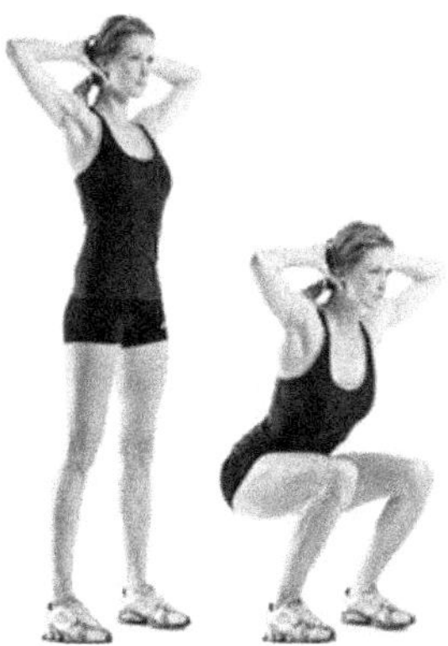

You want to make sure you are sinking your bottom back and not pushing your knees forward. Never put your knees over your toes, this is really hard for your knees.

Keep the move slow and deliberate, controlled weight movement does a lot more for your body than popping in and out of the movement quickly.

Military presses

Stand up tall, and raise one leg until you have your knee bent at a right angle. You are going to be standing on one foot for this, so if you need to hang onto something at first feel free.

However, the stronger you get, the easier it is going to be to hold onto the move without hanging onto anything. When you are able to stand on one foot easily, lift your elbows out to the side so they are at right angles.

Now, raise your hands up over your head while lifting your foot at the same time. Your foot should be out as far as you can get it when your hands are directly above your head.

Slowly bring your hands back down to your elbows being at a right angle, as you slowly lower your foot until your knee is also at a right angle. This is a single military press. Repeat as many times as you can for the duration of your set.

Chair squats

Keep your feet considerably closer together than if you were doing a regular squat. Sit your butt back directly behind you, lowering your knees into a right angle.

Make sure you keep your knees back; you never want them to come over your knees. It is very bad for your knees to push them forward over your toes when you are in a squat.

Sit back as far as you can, slowly, and then stand back up. Squeeze your butt together when you stand up, pressing your pelvis forward. Keep this contraction on your bottom for a full second, then release and sit back again into your chair sit once more.

These are chair squats.

Chapter 3 – Any Day is Leg Day: Leg Exercises for Flexible Toning

We all want to have those nice, toned thighs and that firm, shapely backside. The problem is the more cardio you get, the harder it is to get those toned lower parts. This is because your body likes to store fat for cardio more than it does muscle, so you are going to have to work extra hard if you want to have those thighs and that butt.

You can do these workouts either standing still or moving, you will get the same results either way, but be careful. Leg workouts and the lower body workouts are the ones that tend to cause the most injuries because people tend to stretch too far or push themselves too hard.

You need to listen to your body and pay attention to how far you can comfortably move. If you feel strain or like you are about to hurt yourself, you need to slow down and ease up. It isn't worth an injury to push yourself a little further. You will build up to it, you just have to get there slowly.

The good news is, none of these moves are difficult to execute, they are just difficult to keep doing. You will see that your legs get tired quickly and easily, so work at them for a while and you will see yourself get stronger.

Plank jacks

Lift yourself into a plank, with your back flat, your hands directly beneath you facing forward, and lifted onto the balls of your feet.

Now, jump a powerful jump (as long as you are firmly planted on your hands) and spread your feet out to either side as you reach the jack. You are going to be doing the same thing as you would if you were doing jumping jacks, but you will be down in a plank position.

Keep your bottom at the same level when you are on the inward part of your plank jack, you don't want you bottom to sink down as this could cause strain on your back. Keep your abs strong the entire time you are jumping.

Static lunges with rows

Sink down directly towards the floor, a straight line from the top of your head down to the floor. You want your back to be flat as and your shoulders up.

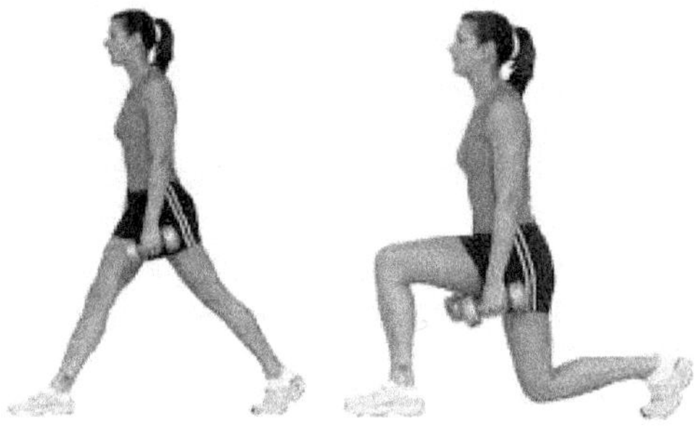

Place one foot forward. For the sake of the example I will say your right foot, although it doesn't matter if it is your right foot or left foot.

Keep your front leg bent at a right angle. You don't want your knee to come over your toe, this is really bad for your knee. Keep it at a right angle.

Keep both feet planted on the floor, with your back leg straight. You will be pretty low to the ground with this.

Place your hands in front of you with your shoulders up, your palms facing each other. Draw your arms back, pinching your shoulders together, holding your stomach in the entire time.

You want this to be a very tight pose.

Jumping lunges

Sink down directly towards the floor, a straight line from the top of your head down to the floor. You want your back to be flat as and your shoulders up.

Place one foot forward. For the sake of the example I will say your right foot, although it doesn't matter if it is your right foot or left foot.

Keep your front leg bent at a right angle. You don't want your knee to come over your toe, this is really bad for your knee. Keep it at a right angle.

Keep both feet planted on the floor, with your back leg straight. You will be pretty low to the ground with this.

Next, launch yourself out of the lunge and jump up into the air. Switch your legs in the air, and land your pose firmly, before sinking back down into a lunge on the other side.

It is very important that you can switch your legs in the air without tripping, and that you stick your landing before you sink down again. There are a lot of injuries that happen to people that aren't capable of doing an exercise and attempting it anyway.

Only do what you know you can do, and build up to a confident level.

Rock Star jumps

Stand up straight, and jump up as high as you can. As you jump, kick both of your legs back as quickly as you can, bending your knees back. You are going to do this so quickly that you jump back and bend both of your knees, then you land back on your feet once more.

As you jump and bend your knees, raise your hands in the air with your elbows bent at a right angle. You can swing your arms down as you land and bend your knees into a deep squat.

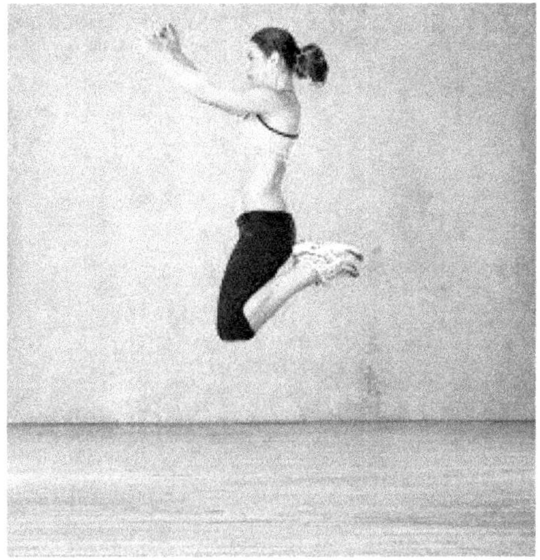

Leap out of your squat and launch into the air while kicking your legs back behind you at the same time and raising your arms at the same time.

These are rock star jumps.

Static Squats and rows

Start by standing with your feet slightly more than hip width apart. Sink your bottom back behind you, sitting down into a squat. Hold your stomach in and keep it firm the entire time, your back flat, and your head up.

Keep your knees at right angles, but make sure your knees never come over your toes as you are sitting. This is very bad for your knees and we don't want any injuries.

Stay here, and keep your shoulders up, push your hands forward, your palms down. Then pull them back again, pinching your shoulders together the entire time.

Make sure as you are doing this that you stay down in a squat the entire time. As you get tired, you will be tempted to stand up out of the squat, sometimes without even realizing that you are.

If you notice yourself standing up, simply sink back down into your squat once more.

Backward leg lifts

Get into a plank pose, on the balls of your feet with your back flat and your bottom even where it should be. Don't lift your bottom up or let it sink down.

Keep your shoulders even and solid, and your hands directly down in front of you, your hands facing forward.

Now, lift one leg off the ground and press your heel into the sky. Pinch your bottom as you get it to the tallest part you can, then slowly lower your foot back down.

Repeat this with the other foot. Hold your stomach firm the entire time, and make sure you maintain your plank pose.

Donkey kicks

Start on your hands and knees, keeping your back flat the entire time. Keep your hands pressed firmly on the floor, and keep your stomach firm.

Now, lift your foot up to the sky, keeping your leg bent. Your knee is going to stay at a right angle the entire time you are doing the move.

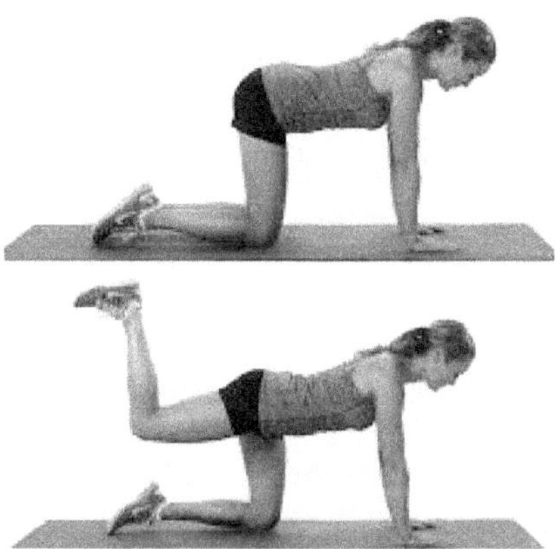

Switch to the other foot, and repeat until you are done with the set.

Sideways lunges with arm lifts

Stand with your feet at a nice wide stance. Lean over to one side, and as you do, let your bottom go out and back. You are going to bend your knee at a right angle on the side you are bending.

You want to sink out and back, never pushing that knee over the toes. This is really bad for your knee and will cause strain on your leg.

As you are sinking back, your other foot is going to stay firm on the floor. Never roll your foot in, this could cause all kinds of injuries. As you are sinking back, keep your shoulders firm, your stomach pulled in at the belly button, and lifting both of your arms.

Your palms will be faced down, and you only bring them up to eye level. Then drop them down again. As you are lifting and dropping into your lunge, you need to time it so you are in a single, uniform flow.

If you do this correctly, you will feel it in your bottom, your shoulders, your upper arms, and your inner thigh. There won't be any strain anywhere, and you will feel your heart rate rise.

Practice to make this move as smooth as possible.

Butt kicks

Start by standing with your feet a little wider than hip width apart. You are going to do an exaggerated version of running in place. As you run, lift your foot as high as you can, literally kicking yourself in the butt with each step.

You will obviously have to almost jump a little with each step, so make sure you don't land on your foot the wrong way and twist it. Keep your arms bent and engaged, you can lower and raise them for extra benefit, or you can just keep them up at your side as though you were jogging in place.

Chapter 4 – Abs of Steel

It seems as though abs are the favorite part of most bodies. We all focus on working those abs, showing off those abs, and tightening those abs. That is the very reason I have included all of these ab workouts. Each of them will tone your abs and build that six pack you have always wanted.

You know you want to wear that swimsuit at the pool and feel great as you do it. If you focus on your abs often, you will see the results of your hard work. Just keep in mind that it takes a little while for abs to show, but as soon as you start to see the results, you will feel even more motivated to stick with it.

These workouts are set up to fit within 10 minutes of time, but you will get results faster if you continue to work your abs for as long as you can do the move properly. Let go of the pose when you can't do it the right way any longer, and you will see your abs grow in strength.

Sit ups

Lay on your back with your knees bent. Your feet will be flat on the floor. Place your fingers behind your ears. You are probably used to clasping them behind your neck, but this is a very bad idea as it can cause a lot of strain on your neck.

Keep your fingertips just behind your ears, not pulling on your head at all. Keep your eyes on the ceiling as you raise yourself up, pushing your throat up to the ceiling with each lift. Stop when you are up in a sitting position, and lower yourself back down.

Slow and controlled.

Crunches

Lay on your back with your knees bent. Your feet will be flat on the floor. Place your fingers behind your ears. You are probably used to clasping them behind your neck, but this is a very bad idea as it can cause a lot of strain on your neck.

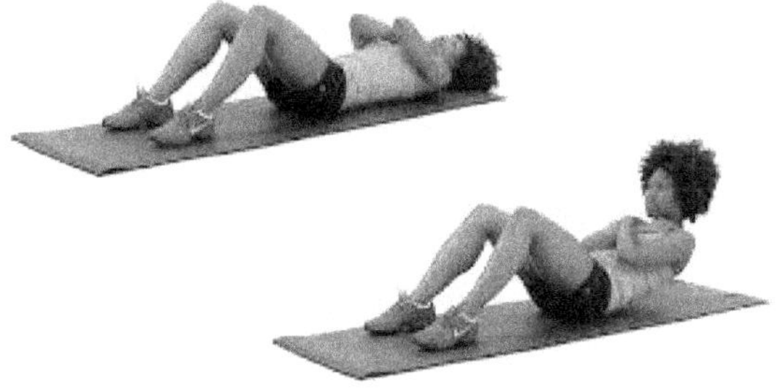

Lift your chest off the floor, eyes on the ceiling and pushing your throat up. No strain on the neck or head. Lift as high as you can, keeping your lower back on the floor, then lower down again.

Reverse crunches

Lay flat on your back with your hands flat on the floor, your arms down at your side. Lift your legs up and bend your knees, so your knees are at a right angle.

Next, roll your bottom up off the floor, lifting just your bottom up off the floor. Raise it as high as you can, then lower it again. Slow and controlled deliberate.

Pipe crunches

Lay on your back with your arms outstretched, also on the floor. Your legs are to also be outstretched on the floor in front of you.

Lift both your hands and your feet at the same time, keeping your arms and legs straight on the way up, pressing into a crunch at the top. You want to inhale on your way down, exhale on your way up. Exhale as much as possible at the top, getting as much of a crunch as possible.

Bicycle crunches

Lay on your back with your knees bent. Your feet will be flat on the floor. Place your fingers behind your ears. You are probably used to clasping them behind your neck, but this is a very bad idea as it can cause a lot of strain on your neck.

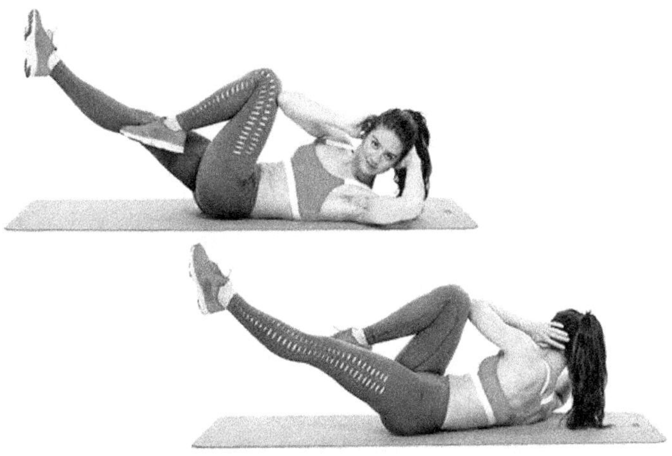

With each raise of your shoulders, pull one knee in and extend your other leg out. As you alternate, alternate your shoulders. Think of it as riding a bicycle only you are lying on your back.

Mountain climbers

Settle into a plank pose, with your back flat and your bottom where it should be, not too high and not sunk down. Keep your shoulders even and your arms straight with your hands flat on the floor.

Now, pump your knees inward, and set them back to land on the balls of your feet. Almost like a sprinter getting ready at the starting gate, only never standing up. Keep your movements powerful, pushing those knees in and planting them firmly on your way back out.

You need to keep your abs pulled in at the belly button, tight the entire time even as you get sore when you keep the movement going. Keep it up as long as the duration of your set.

Double crunches

Lay on your back with your knees bent. Your feet will be flat on the floor. Place your fingers behind your ears. You are probably used to clasping them behind your neck, but this is a very bad idea as it can cause a lot of strain on your neck.

Keep your legs up, with your knees bent at a right angle. Lift your bottom up off the floor as you raise your shoulders up off the floor. Inhale when you are lying flat on the floor, and exhale when you are at the peak of your crunch.

Squeeze as firmly as you can while you're lifted off the floor, then release as you lie back. Repeat as many times as you can in a single session.

Scissor kicks

Lay on your back with your hands and arms flat on the floor. Lift your feet up off the floor a few inches with your legs straight.

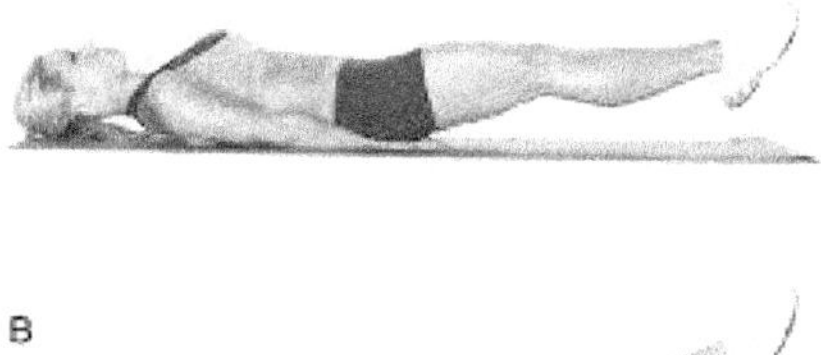

Cross your legs back and forth in a slow and deliberate manner. If you want to make this move a little bit more of a challenge, lift your shoulders up off the floor a few inches as well.

Hold your feet up for the entire duration of the session.

High knees

High knees is an activity that is high energy. You need to do this in shoes or barefoot, but don't do it in socks as you may fall.

Stand with your feet about hip width apart, and hold your hands up and engaged. This means you want your arms bent at a right angle the entire time you are doing the move.

As you do this, you want to raise your knees as high as you can, then barely land on the ground before you raise your other leg as high as you can. Think of it as almost jumping from foot to foot.

Keep this movement fast and steady for as long as the duration of your session.

Chapter 5 – The Upper Body: Strength Training

We all tend to focus on our abs more than anything. When we see the ads and commercials on the television and the magazines, we see the people with washboard abs and tight pecs. They always have the greatest physique all over, but what we see are the abs.

The issue with this is if you were to erase the toning of the rest of the body, and all you could see where the abs, you would find that the entire body would look off. This is why you need to work your arms and legs as much as you do your abs.

These are all workouts that will work your upper body. Your biceps, shoulders, triceps, and back are all the targets of these workouts, and you can do them anytime, anywhere.

Bicep curls

Pull your elbows back so they are firmly against your sides. You are going to bend your arms at right angles when you are extended, but besides that you are going to raise your arms up.

Hold weights in your hands, palms up. Lift your hands at the same time, about three quarters of the way up. Lower them down until your arms are lengthened.

Repeat pulling your hands up then lowering them again, slow and steady the entire time. Control is the name of the game.

Triceps pulses

Stand with your feet hip width apart, and bend at the waist. Bend straight down, keeping your back flat the entire time.

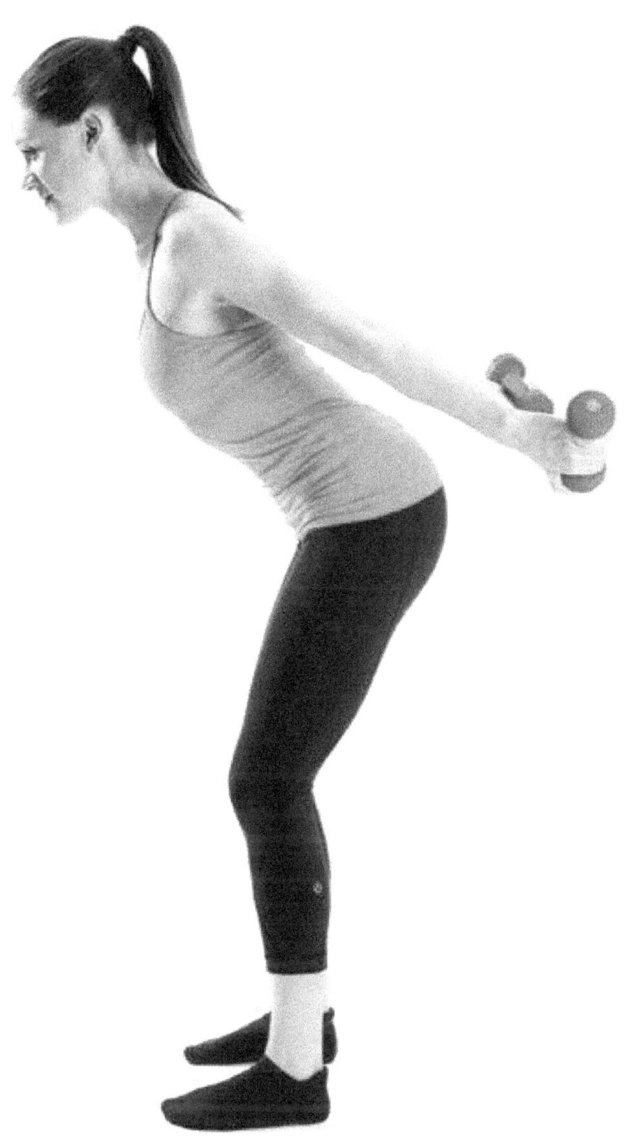

Hold your arms back, keeping them straight. Lift your hands as high as you comfortably can then lower them down again. Pulse this way for the duration of your session, making sure you don't strain too far.

Be careful with this move, you can overdo very easily, and that is going to result in injury for your arms. Make sure you only move as far as is comfortable but still a challenge, working your muscles but not over straining.

Plank jumps

By now you should have your plank pretty well down. Stand on the balls of your feet with your back flat, and your hands flat on the floor. Your arms are going to be straight, so you look very straight when viewed from the side.

For your plank jump, you need to have your hands firmly on the floor, making sure you don't roll your arms one way or the other when you are jumping.

Jump both feet in at the same time, landing about the midpoint of your chest on the floor. Jump them back out again, then back in again. Keep your abs firm, with your belly button pulled in firmly the entire time.

Keep your jumps steady and your head up, so you don't knee yourself in the face.

Keep your feet down so you don't twist them when you land. Stay steady and firm the entire time you do this move.

Triceps raises

Stand with your feet hip width apart, and bend at the waist. Keep your back entirely flat, and pull your abs in.

Keep your head looking down, you don't want to add any strain to your neck.

Place your arms straight down, then pull your elbows up so your arms are bent at a right angle, with your hands down towards the floor.

Extend your arms so your hand lifts, and you can feel the growing tension on your arm, right where your triceps is.

Lower and raise, repeating for as long as your session is. Keep your movement steady and even, not rushing the movement or loosening up at all.

Superman bends

Lay face down on the floor, with your feet on your toes and your arms outstretched over your head, your palms on the floor.

With each raise, life your hands up off the floor, and your knees at the same time. As you lift, pinch your shoulder blades together and pinch your butt cheeks together at the same time.

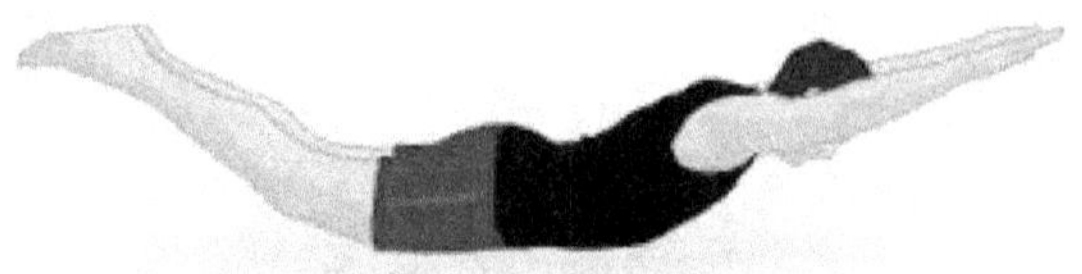

You need to make sure not to lift too high with your legs as you can add strain to the back of your thighs, just lift as much as is comfortable, yet provides a challenge.

In other words, don't lift until you strain, just lift enough that you are adding tension to the back of your leg. You will feel this in your bottom, your back, and your shoulders if you are doing this the right way.

Lift and lower in a slow and steady way for the duration of your session.

Punches

Lower down into a squat, with your feet a little wider than your hips. You want to get as low into your squat as you can, but never push your knees over your toes, this is really bad for your knees.

Punch the air, stretching your arms across your body so you can feel it in your back, and so you get a nice rotation in your torso. Keep your torso upright, you don't want to slouch, even though you are in a squat.

Punch as quickly as you can, keeping your pace even and timing your breathing with each of your punches. This will raise your heart rate faster than anything else.

Chest flies

Lay on your back with your knees bent and your feet flat on the floor. Hold weights in both of your hands and lower them down to the ground, palms up.

Raise them again over your chest, making sure to keep them over your chest and not over your stomach or over your head. Right over your chest is the perfect spot for this move.

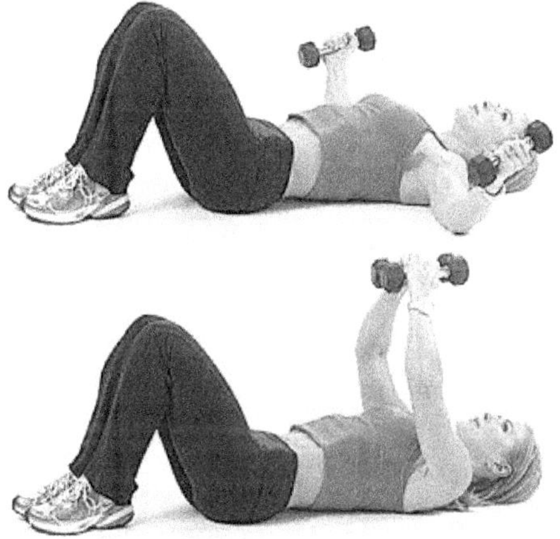

Raise and lower for the duration of your session.

Burpees

Start standing up, then drop down to a hunched position. Jump your feet back to a plank, then jump back forward to your hunched position.

From there, jump up as high as you can from the crouch, then land and crouch down again. Jump back to your plank, then jump up.

Repeat as many of these as you can for the duration of your set.

Oblique Twists with weights

Hold weights in both of your hands, and twist your body so your head and shoulders are the opposite direction of the way your feet are pointing. Jump up, and twist your torso and your feet so your body is in the opposite positon as they were when you started.

Jump this way back and forth for as long as your session, keeping your arms up to shoulder height for the entire duration of the exercise. Make sure your arms are up, you don't want to let them droop down as you get tired.

Chapter 6 – Bringing it all Together: Full Body Workouts

You need to focus on each part of your body at some point throughout the week, and it is important that you work in plenty of cardio throughout your workout, but every now and then, you also have to just work your entire body.

These are the workouts that work everything. Not too much focus on any one part, but plenty of work for your entire body. If you do any of these workouts, you will get an all over toning that shows off your whole hot self.

Warm up

For your warm up, start with arm crosses. Hold your arms out to the side, and cross them over each other, then open up, and cross them over each other once more.

Each time you cross over, make sure the opposite arm is on top than the first cross. Do this for 10 seconds.

Next, do a set of jumping jacks for another 20 seconds. I assume you already know how to do a jumping jack, so I won't describe that one.

Next, do a few leg kicks. Start by kicking low, then gradually raise your leg higher and higher as you kick. Keep the kicks slow and deliberate. Do this for 20 seconds.

Finally, do one more set of arm crosses for a final 10 seconds, and you are warmed up for your workout.

Full Body Workout 1

Squat low with weights in your hand, then stand up. Repeat this for 30 seconds. Switch from this to plank jacks for another 30 seconds. Go back to the squats for another 30 seconds, and finish with another 30 seconds of plank jacks.

Get down on the floor and work your abs with sit ups for a minute straight. Get up and do a set of butt kicks for 30 seconds, then jumping jacks for 30 seconds. Do this set once more, then get back on the floor for bicycle crunches for 1 minute.

Flip over and do push-ups for 30 seconds, then slow mountain climbers for another 30 seconds. Go back to the 30 seconds of push-ups, then the mountain climbers for another 30 seconds.

Get up off the floor and do a set of jumping jacks for a minute straight, then finish with a set of crunches for 30 seconds, then reverse crunches for your final 30 seconds.

That's it! Workout 1 complete in 10 minutes.

Full Body Workout 2

After your warm up, start out strong with a set of jumping jacks, hard and strong for 1 minute straight. Get down on the floor and do as many push-ups as you can in another minute.

From there, roll over on your back and do bicycle crunches for another minute, then get up again and do another set of jumping jacks for another minute. I know your heart is going to be racing right now, but you need to push forward and switch to weight training to bring down your heart rate.

Grab your weights, and do a set of military presses first on your right leg for 30 seconds, then switch to your left leg for the other 30 seconds. You are now half-way through your workout.

Get down on the floor, and do a set of chest flies for 30 seconds. Stop with your hands over your chest with your weights in your hand, and do a set of reverse crunches for another minute, then set down your weights and roll back over on your front.

Lift yourself in a plank, and hold your plank for an entire minute. Drop down to your knees, and alternate your legs as you do donkey kicks for 1 minute, alternating your legs each time.

Stand up, then sink down into a squat, and air box for 30 seconds. Do a last set of jumping jacks for another minute.

That's it! That's the end of workout 2. Make sure you bring your heart rate back down with the cool down before you get back to the rest of your day.

Full Body Workout 3

After your warm up, drop down to a plank, and do as many mountain climbers as fast as you can for an entire minute. Stand up and do high knees as fast as you can for another minute, then switch to butt kicks for another minute.

Your heart is going to be racing by this time, so grab your weights. Stand with your feet slightly wider than your hips, and do dead lifts for 30 seconds. Roll over on your back, and do a set of sit ups for 30 seconds.

Lay back, and hold your feet down over the ground, about 2 inches up off the floor. Proceed to do scissor kicks for another minute.

Stand up and repeat another set of jumping jacks for another minute, then drop to the floor and do another set of push-ups for 30 seconds. Pull your arms in and repeat another set of mountain climbers for another 30 seconds.

After your mountain climbers, stretch out in a full plank position, and alternate lifting each leg for a minute, then drop down onto your stomach and do superman lifts for another minute.

Do these lifts slow and steady, raising both knees and your arms off the floor at the same time.

Stand up and do a set of butt kicks for 30 seconds, then switch to high knees for another 30 seconds.

That's it! That's the end of the workout 3, but you are going to end with your heart racing, so you need to make sure you do the cool down before you get back to the rest of your day.

Cool down

Complete your final minute of working out, and walk around for 20 seconds. When you feel your heart rate return down to a more normal rate, sit down into a sitting split as far as you comfortably can. Reach one arm up and over the top of your head, and gently pull it further down with your other arm.

Repeat this on the other side, stretching out your other arm. Stand up and put your hands on the wall, pushing against the wall, with your feet planted securely on the floor.

Lean into the stretch, stretching out your hamstrings. Lean as far down as you can without putting too much stress on your lower legs. Stand up, and grab your left foot with your left hand. Pull your heel into the back of your leg, careful not to pull your foot out from your body, as this will add strain to your knee.

If you need to hang onto something for balance, try standing close to a chair or the back of a couch to stabilize yourself as you stretch out your leg. Repeat this on the other side, stretching each leg for 10 to 15 seconds.

Mix and match!

You are free to mix and match the exercises that are in the workouts, and you can combine the workouts to make them longer if you want. I can't stress enough how important it is for you to warm up and cool down for each one, but you can do 1, 2, or even all three of the workouts at once if you want to.

There's nothing wrong with doing just one, and you are more than welcome to do more than that if you want. You aren't going to work out too much if you do more than the one, but you aren't going to miss out on the benefits if you only do the one, too.

I want you to have fun with this and enjoy the process as much as you like the results, so if you want to work out more because you like it, then you should! But if you only work out so you can get the benefits, you will get them if you only do the single work outs.

Also keep in mind you can mix and match the workouts by mixing up the workout you do for the length of time. For instance, you can change out pull ups for the push-ups in the workouts, and you can do more or less cardio if you like.

My point is you are going to get excellent results no matter what your workout is, as long as you are doing a mix of muscle, cardio, and abs.

Have fun and relax with your workouts, and fall in love with the results that you earn in no time at all.

Insider's tip:

So many people feel as though they can skip the warm up and the cool down to their workouts. Especially when they aren't working out for very long. While you can survive without warming up or cooling down, you aren't going to get the same kind of benefits if you do.

Stretching after a workout is what helps your muscles regain their elasticity and grow stronger. On the other hand, if you skip out on the warm up, you are risking injury by working muscles that aren't loose or ready to work.

It only takes a few minutes to do the war up and cool down combined, so take the extra seconds to save yourself the soreness and potential injury later on in your day. A few seconds now is always better than the hours of recovery you would face if you injured yourself.

Chapter 7 – Game Plan Level: Fit

There are a number of workouts you have to choose from now, but you can't just pick the ones you like and ignore the others. As you saw in the last chapters, it is important to work out each part of your body specifically on different days, because you will lose out on the hard work you have done if you don't.

The more you use the parts of your body, the more you are going to see the results you want to see. I have now put together a plan for you to follow with these workouts I have provided above.

This is a 10 day plan, so if you stick with it, you will be able to get through the entire thing 3 times in a month. I know it will be a bit of a shock for you when you get to day 10 and you see that you are supposed to take a day off, but let me assure you, I know what I am doing.

The reason there is a day off 3 times a month is dual-purpose. First of all, you need to recover. Our bodies weren't designed to go at it for that level of intensity every day, even if it isn't all day. Secondly, I want you to see that you can take a day off and things are going to be all right.

Too many people think if they ever take a day off that it will all fall apart and they won't reach their goals, but since you can see that you are deliberately taking days off, you know it is just fine for you to still reach your goals.

Day 1

Warm up, Full Body Workout 1, cool down

Day 2 – leg day

Warm up, static lunge and row for 2 minutes, 1 minute per side. Follow this with walking lunges for 1 minute. Squat and lift weights for another minute, complete a set of jumping jacks for 1 minute, then finish with planking for a full minute. Do a set of jumping jacks for another minute, then drop down to a plank and do leg raises for another full minute. Roll over on your back, and do reverse crunches for a final minute. Cool down

Day 3- upper body

Warm up, then get right down to it with an entire minute of jumping jacks. Drop down to the floor and do a set of push-ups for 30 seconds. Place your hands beneath you in a plank, and finish out the minute with 30 seconds of plank jacks.

Flip over on your back, and do a set of chest flies for 30 seconds. When you reach the 30 seconds, keep your hands up and over your chest, then lift one leg off the floor, and drop it again, then repeat on the other side. Do this for 30 seconds, alternating each leg.

Get back up, with a weight in each hand, and hold your hands out to the side. Begin doing oblique twists, and hold this for 30 seconds. Set down your weights and go back to jumping jacks for the rest of the 30 seconds in that minute.

Grab both of your weights, and drop down into a squat. Hold the squat as long as you can, or pop in and out of the squat if your legs aren't strong enough yet to hold the squat for the full 30 seconds. As you are in your squat, keep a weight in each hand and do bicep curls as you are in and out of your squat. Next, bend forward, and hold your hands behind you and pulse your hands up with the weights. This is going to work out your triceps.

You are halfway through your workout now.

Launch your heart rate back up with 30 seconds of air boxing, and finish the minute with 30 seconds of jumping jacks.

Drop down to the floor, and do a set of sit ups for another minute. Lay back on the floor and repeat reverse crunches for 30 seconds, then go to double crunches for 30 seconds.

Roll back over onto your stomach and life yourself into a plank. Do another set of push-ups for 30 seconds, then plank jacks for another 30 seconds. Get up and finish strong with your last minute of jumping jacks. Cool down

Day 4 – ab and body weight

Warm up, then launch your heart rate with a nice set of high knees. I want these to be powerful for the entire minute as you lift your knees up into the air for 1 minute. Leave your high knees and embrace a set of jumping jacks for another minute.

Drop down to your plank, and slowly do a set of push-ups for 30 seconds, then raise your legs alternately for the last 30 seconds. Roll onto your back, and do reverse crunches for 30 seconds, then regular crunches for 30 seconds.

Now, lay both of your hands up behind you and your legs out flat, and do pipe crunches for 30 seconds, then finish it out with bicycle crunches for 30 seconds.

You have reached the half-way point of your workout.

Stand up, and do a full minute of military presses, 30 seconds on each foot, then get back on the floor and do another minute of side raises, 30 seconds on each side.

Lay face down on your stomach, and do a set of superman raises for one minute, then get up again and do another minute of high knees. Drop down onto the floor once more, and plank for your last minute. Cool down

Day 5

Warm up, Full Body Workout 2, cool down

Day 6 – leg day

Warm up, jump in with 1 minute of butt kicks.

Drop down to the floor and do plank jacks for 30 seconds, then bring your heart rate down with 30 seconds of donkey kicks.

Drop further down onto your stomach and engage in superman lifts for 1 minute. Come back up into your plank and alternate leg lifts for another minute. Launch your heart rate with mountain climbers for another minute, then slowly do push-ups for 30 seconds.

Hold a straight plank for 30 seconds. You are now half-way through your workout.

Stand up and grab your weights, then sink down and slowly come up out of squats for 30 seconds. Set down your weights and do a set of alternating jumping lunges for another 30 seconds.

Drop down into a static lunge and row with your left leg forward for 30 seconds, then switch legs for another 30 seconds. Bring your heart rate up with another minute of butt kicks, and sink into a low squat for 30 seconds of punches.

Drop down and do another set of push-ups for 30 seconds, then finish with one full minute of alternating back leg lifts. Cool down

Day 7 – upper body

Warm up, begin by bringing your heart rate up with a full minute of jumping jacks, then work your obliques in there with 30 seconds of oblique twists. Drop down and do plank jacks for 30 seconds, then switch it up with 30 seconds of plank jumps.

Roll over on your back, and grab your weights. Slowly do a set of chest flies for 30 seconds, then drop your weights and do a full minute of sit-ups. Roll back onto your stomach, and do a full minute of slow push-ups.

You are at the half-way point of your workout.

Drop down into a low squat, and punch the air as quickly as you can for another minute, launching your heart rate. Grab your weights once more and do a set of military presses with your weights, 30 seconds on each side for 1 minute total. Drop down into a static lunge and row for 30 seconds, then move to your other leg forward and row for another 30 seconds. Come out of your lunges and do a set of dead lifts for 30 seconds, then bring your heart rate back up with a set of oblique twists with weights for 30 seconds.

Drop to your back and do a set of sit-ups for 30 seconds, then lie back and finish your last 30 seconds with a set of chest flies. Cool down

Day 8 – abs and body weight

Warm up, then start with a full minute of hard jumping jacks. Lay down on your back, and do a set of bicycle crunches for another minute. Roll onto your stomach, and do a full minute of push-ups, strong and quickly.

Stand back up, and do a set of walking lunges for 30 seconds, then do a set of military presses for 30 seconds, 15 seconds on each side. Drop down into a plank, and launch your heart rate with mountain climbers for a full minute, then switch to 30 seconds of plank jumps, and bring your heart rate back down with 30 seconds of planking.

Roll onto your back, and do a set of double crunches for a full minute. Grab your weights, and do a set of chest flies for 30 seconds, then roll onto your stomach and finish the minute with superman lifts.

Pull yourself up into a plank, and do a set of push-ups for 30 seconds, then plank for 30 seconds.

Stand up and do a fast and furious set of high knees for your last minute. Cool down.

Day 9

Warm up, Full Body Workout 3, cool down

Day 10

Take a day off. Seriously, you deserve it.

Now, you need to run through this set of workouts during your month, but feel free to mix and match the exact workouts you are doing. For example, if you see that day 2 is ab day, do an ab workout, but don't feel like you always have to do the same ab move.

The more you work different parts of your body, the better the results you are going to see. Maybe do crunches one day, then reverse crunches the next time you do abs. Then go back to crunches when you get ab day again.

The more moves you know, the more you can mix it up, and the more diversity you will get with the moves on that particular part of your body. This, in turn, is going to lead to better results as well.

When you know how to work out smart, you reach your goals faster, and you see better results than you would if you were stuck in the old school way of doing things.

Bonus – Meal Plan to Jumps Start Your Success

If you want to lose weight and keep it off, and if you want to lose weight the safe and healthy way, you have to combine it with a meal plan. It is a myth if you cut out all of the food besides broccoli and spinach you aren't going to reach your goals, but it is just as much a myth that you can live off of pizza and ice cream and still hope to reach them.

Either way you look at it, you have to give in and compromise somewhere. Now, I have never been one for total deprivation. I think that sets you up for failure, and only starts the clock to the point when you will cave in and binge on exactly what you shouldn't.

Don't believe me? Well, give it a try and let me know how long that lasts. On the other hand, if you let yourself have some of the food that you do love, even the food that isn't healthy, you will be a lot more likely to stick with your meal plan as a whole and get better results.

The reason this is true is because high intensity interval training revs up your metabolism, so even if you aren't burning hundreds of calories in a workout, you are making your body use the energy you put into it more efficiently. That means you lose weight faster, even working out less.

That's enough chit chat. Let's get down to a plan that is going to help you lose the weight and keep it off for good!

Monday

Breakfast – whole grain cereal with milk and a banana

Lunch – pasta salad with chicken cut up into it

Dinner – meat loaf and mashed potatoes

Tuesday

Breakfast – mixed fruit smoothie

Lunch – boiled eggs, nuts, and carrot sticks

Dinner – sausage and rice casserole with veggies

Wednesday

Breakfast – English muffin with fried egg and cheese

Lunch – chicken fajitas

Dinner – turkey meatballs and whole grains

Thursday

Breakfast – oatmeal with fruit and nuts

Lunch – chicken salad

Dinner – Homemade mac n cheese with side of veggies

Friday

Breakfast – whole wheat toast with peanut butter

Lunch – veggie salad and protein of your choice

Dinner – cheat night! Have whatever you want!

Saturday

Breakfast – veggie omelet with cheese

Lunch – chicken breast sandwich and healthy chips

Dinner – taco salad

Sunday

Breakfast – Whole wheat pancake and syrup

Lunch – fruit smoothie made with yogurt, side of nuts

Dinner – pot roast and veggies

You probably noticed that I left the meals themselves pretty open. This is because it doesn't want you to feel like you have to get stuck in a week's worth of meals and feel like you can't eat anything else if you want to lose weight.

You may have also noticed that I didn't measure out the portions for each of the meals, and I also have a reason for that. You see, when you start to obsess over how much of this and how little of that, you are setting yourself up for disaster. The way you live your life is the way you live your life.

I believe if you are working out regularly with these workouts, and you eat the healthy meals like described, you don't have to stress about numbers and measures.

If you stick with the idea of these meals, you are, however, going to have the freedom to choose what you want to eat and still have that ripped, toned body you have been waiting for.

Stick with the workout and stick with the meal plan, and I promise you in no time at all you will start to see the results, and shortly after that you will see the results get better as your body changes and adapts right into what you want it to be.

Good luck!

Conclusion

There you have it, everything you need to know to lose weight and get fit, all from the comfort of your own living room or anywhere else you want to squeeze in a quick workout.

Remember that the next step is to stick with it, and not get discouraged if you want to do something better but aren't there yet. You may find that it takes a little while for you to see the fruit of your labor, but in less than 2 months tops you will see that muscle definition you have been looking for. It doesn't take much for you to get that look you desire, and it takes even less time to keep it.

When you realize how fast and easy it is to lose the weight you want to lose, you are going to wonder why more people don't get out there and do it. It seems too easy not to do, so you wonder why they spend so much time at the gym or doing other things that don't get them nearly the same results.

I want you to succeed at this, so stay positive, and remember that you are incredible no matter what you weigh. Never get stuck in the frame of thought that tells you that you have to weight a certain number or look a certain way in order to be attractive, because you are perfect just like you are.

My goal with this book is to help you gain the confidence you need to strut your stuff and be the beautiful you that you were intended to be. I know you can do it, and I know it won't take nearly as long as you fear it will. If you follow the guides in this book, you will have that definition in less than two months.

That means if you start right now, you will be fit and toned by the time summer gets here, perfect for those bathing suit days.

The new you is about ready for their perfect debut! You just have to let loose and let them out once and for all!

FREE Bonus Reminder

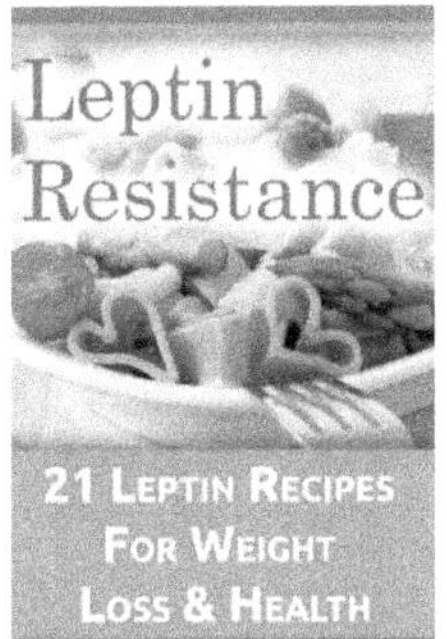

If you have not grabbed it yet, please go ahead and download your special bonus report *"Leptin Resistance. 21 Leptin Recipes For Weight Loss & Healthy Living"*.

Simply Click the Button Below

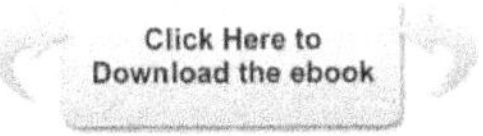

OR **Go to This Page**

http://easyweightlossway.com/free/

BONUS #2: More Free & Discounted Books

Do you want to receive more Free & Discounted Books?

We have a mailing list where we send out our new Books when they go free or with a discount on Kindle. Click on the link below to sign up for Free & Discount Book Promotions.

=> Sign Up for Free & Discount Book Promotions <=

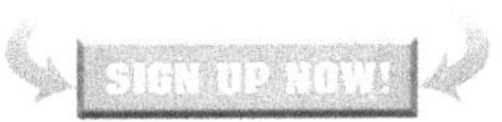

OR Go to this URL

http://zbit.ly/1WBb1Ek